# Endo Wellness

## MANAGING ENDOMETRIOSIS THROUGH DIET, NUTRITION AND REMEDIES

## Dr. Kate Madison

# Copyright


No part of this book should be copied, reproduced without the author's permission @2024 Endo Wellness by Dr. Kate Madison

# TABLE OF CONTENTS

# Introduction

Welcome to Endo Wellness, a comprehensive guide to reclaiming control of your health and vitality in the face of endometriosis. In the landscape of women's health, endometriosis stands as a formidable challenge, affecting millions worldwide with its debilitating symptoms and often elusive solutions. However, within the pages of this book lies a holistic blueprint for managing endometriosis that transcends the limitations of conventional medicine.

At its essence, Endo Wellness embodies a philosophy rooted in empowerment, resilience, and the transformative power of holistic healing. Through a multifaceted approach encompassing diet, nutrition, and natural remedies, we embark on a journey of self-discovery and self-care, illuminating the path towards greater well-being and vitality.

Our journey commences by unraveling the intricate tapestry of endometriosis, from its enigmatic origins to its complex manifestations within the body. Through the lens of science and personal narratives, we explore the myriad factors contributing to this condition, including hormonal imbalances, immune dysfunction, and genetic predispositions.

Central to our approach is the recognition that true healing begins from within. We delve into the profound impact of diet and nutrition on endometriosis, offering evidence-based insights, meal plans, and recipes tailored to support hormonal balance, reduce inflammation, and alleviate symptoms. From anti-inflammatory superfoods to hormone-balancing herbs, we empower you to make informed choices that nourish your body and promote optimal health.

But Endo Wellness extends beyond the realm of nutrition; it encompasses a holistic framework that addresses the mind, body, and spirit in harmony. We explore the transformative power of mindfulness, stress reduction techniques, and mind-body practices in managing pain, enhancing resilience, and fostering emotional well-being.

Furthermore, we delve into the rich tapestry of natural remedies and alternative therapies that have shown promise in alleviating endometriosis symptoms. From herbal supplements and acupuncture to aromatherapy and pelvic physiotherapy, we illuminate the diverse array of holistic modalities available to support your healing journey.

Yet, amidst the wealth of information and guidance, we never lose sight of the individuality of each person's experience with endometriosis. We honor the voices of those who have traversed this path before, sharing their stories of struggle, triumph, and resilience as beacons of inspiration for others.

Endo Wellness is more than just a book; it is a manifesto for reclaiming agency over your health, a roadmap for navigating the complexities of endometriosis, and a testament to the transformative power of holistic healing. Join us as we embark on this empowering journey towards greater vitality, resilience, and well-being.

Endometriosis is a disease in which tissue similar to the lining of the uterus grows outside the uterus. It can cause severe pain in the pelvis and make it harder to get pregnant.

Endometriosis can start at a person's first menstrual period and last until menopause.

With endometriosis, tissue similar to the lining of the uterus grows outside the uterus. This leads to inflammation and scar tissue forming in the pelvic region and (rarely) elsewhere in the body.

The cause of endometriosis is unknown. There is no known way to prevent endometriosis. There is no cure, but its symptoms can be treated with medicines or, in some cases, surgery.

It causes a chronic inflammatory reaction that may result in the formation of scar tissue (adhesions, fibrosis) within the pelvis and other parts of the body. Several lesion types have been described:

- Superficial endometriosis found mainly on the pelvic peritoneum
- Cystic ovarian endometriosis (endometrioma) found in the ovaries
- Deep endometriosis found in the recto-vaginal septum, bladder, and bowel
- In rare cases, endometriosis has also been found outside the pelvis.

# Symptoms

The main symptom of endometriosis is pelvic pain. It's often linked with menstrual periods. Although many people have cramping during their periods, those with endometriosis often describe menstrual pain that's far worse than usual. The pain also may become worse over time.

**Common symptoms of endometriosis include:**

- Painful periods: Pelvic pain and cramping may start before a menstrual period and last for days into it. You also may have lower back and stomach pain. Another name for painful periods is dysmenorrhea.
- Pain with sex: Pain during or after sex is common with endometriosis.
- Pain with bowel movements or urination: You're most likely to have these symptoms before or during a menstrual period.
- Excessive bleeding: Sometimes, you may have heavy menstrual periods or bleeding between periods.
- Infertility: For some people, endometriosis is first found during tests for infertility treatment.

- Other symptoms: You may have fatigue, diarrhea, constipation, bloating or nausea. These symptoms are more common before or during menstrual periods.

The seriousness of your pain may not be a sign of the number or extent of endometriosis growths in your body. You could have a small amount of tissue with bad pain. Or you could have lots of endometriosis tissue with little or no pain.

Still, some people with endometriosis have no symptoms. Often, they find out they have the condition when they can't get pregnant or after they get surgery for another reason.

For those with symptoms, endometriosis sometimes may seem like other conditions that can cause pelvic pain. These include pelvic inflammatory disease or ovarian cysts. Or it may be confused with irritable bowel syndrome (IBS), which causes bouts of diarrhea, constipation and stomach cramps. IBS also can happen along with endometriosis. This makes it harder for your health care team to find the exact cause of your symptoms.

# Diagnosis

It can be difficult for a medical professional to diagnose endometriosis because no specific test can confirm it, and the symptoms may be hard to see. The symptoms can also resemble the symptoms of other conditions.

Possible diagnostic strategies include|:

- Apelvic exam
- Imaging tests, such as an ultrasound or MRI scan
- Laparoscopy
- A biopsy

Surgical laparoscopy is the only way to confirm a diagnosis of endometriosis. This is a minimally invasive procedure in which a doctor inserts a laparoscope through a small incision in the pelvic area. This provides images of tissue changes.

## When to see a doctor

See a member of your health care team if you think you might have symptoms of endometriosis.

Endometriosis can be a challenge to manage. You may be better able to take charge of the symptoms if:

- Your care team finds the disease sooner rather than later.
- You learn as much as you can about endometriosis.
- You get treatment from a team of health care professionals from different medical fields, if needed.

# Chapter 1

# Understanding endometriosis

**What Is Endometriosis?**

Endometriosis is a common condition in women. It's chronic, it's painful, and it often gets steadily worse.

Normally, the tissue that lines a woman's uterus, known as the endometrium, is found only in the uterus. But when a woman develops endometriosis, microscopic bits of this tissue grow on other organs such as the ovaries, the outer wall of the uterus, the fallopian tubes, the ligaments that support the uterus, the space between the uterus and the rectum, and the space between the uterus and the bladder. In rare cases, they can spread outside the abdomen and grow on other organs, such as the lungs.

Just like the endometrium, the tissue responds to the hormones estrogen and progesterone by thickening, and it may bleed intermittently. But because the tissue is growing in other tissues, the blood it makes cannot escape. This causes irritation to the surrounding tissue, which causes cysts, scars, and the fusing of body tissues. This can eventually bind the reproductive organs together and lead to infertility.

Cases of endometriosis are classified as minimal, mild, moderate, or severe, depending on the size of the lesions and how deeply they reach into the other organs. They are also referred to as stage I-IV.

Endometriosis affects 3% to 10% of women of reproductive age, and 25% to 50% of infertile women. It affects about 40% to 80% of women with pelvic pain. It affects all races equally. Symptoms usually get better after menopause.

## Causes and complications

### Causes

The exact cause of endometriosis isn't clear. But some possible causes include:

- Retrograde menstruation: This is when menstrual blood flows back through the fallopian tubes and into the pelvic cavity instead of out of the body. The blood contains endometrial cells from the inner lining of the uterus. These cells may stick to the pelvic walls and surfaces of pelvic organs. There, they might grow and continue to thicken and bleed over the course of each menstrual cycle.

- Transformed peritoneal cells: Experts suggest that hormones or immune factors might help transform cells that line the inner side of the abdomen, called peritoneal cells, into cells that are like those that line the inside of the uterus.
- Embryonic cell changes: Hormones such as estrogen may transform embryonic cells — cells in the earliest stages of development — into endometrial-like cell growths during puberty.
- Surgical scar complication: Endometrial cells may attach to scar tissue from a cut made during surgery to the stomach area, such as a C-section.
- Endometrial cell transport: The blood vessels or tissue fluid system may move endometrial cells to other parts of the body.

- Immune system condition: A problem with the immune system may make the body unable to recognize and destroy endometriosis tissue.

**Risk factors**

Factors that raise the risk of endometriosis include:

- Never giving birth.
- Starting your period at an early age.
- Going through menopause at an older age.
- Short menstrual cycles — for instance, less than 27 days.
- Heavy menstrual periods that last longer than seven days.
- Having higher levels of estrogen in your body or a greater lifetime exposure to estrogen your body produces.
- Low body mass index.
- One or more relatives with endometriosis, such as a mother, aunt or sister.

Any health condition that prevents blood from flowing out of the body during menstrual periods also can be an endometriosis risk factor. So can conditions of the reproductive tract.

Endometriosis symptoms often happen years after menstruation starts. The symptoms may get better for a time with pregnancy. Pain may become milder over time with menopause, unless you take estrogen therapy.

## Complications

Women with endometriosis can sometimes experience a number of complications.

### Infertility

The main complication of endometriosis is trouble getting pregnant, also called infertility. Up to half of people with endometriosis have a hard time conceiving.

For pregnancy to happen, an egg must be released from an ovary. Then the egg has to travel through the fallopian tube and become fertilized by a sperm cell. The fertilized egg then needs to attach itself to the wall of the uterus to start developing. Endometriosis may block the tube and keep the egg and sperm from uniting. But the condition also seems to affect fertility in less-direct ways. For instance, it may damage the sperm or egg.

Even so, many with mild to moderate endometriosis can still conceive and carry a pregnancy to term. Health care professionals sometimes advise those with endometriosis not to delay having children. That's because the condition may become worse with time.

**Treatment**

There are 3 main types of fertility treatment:

- Medicines
- Surgical procedures
- Assisted conception – including intrauterine insemination (IUI) and in vitro fertilisation (IVF)

**Medicines**

Common fertility medicines include:

- Clomifene – encourages the monthly release of an egg (ovulation) in women who do not ovulate regularly or cannot ovulate at all
- Tamoxifen – an alternative to clomifene that may be offered if you have ovulation problems

- Metformin – is particularly beneficial for women who have polycystic ovary syndrome (PCOS)
- Gonadotrophins – can help stimulate ovulation in women, and may also improve fertility in men
- Gonadotrophin-releasing hormone and dopamine agonists – other types of medicine prescribed to encourage ovulation in women

Some of these medicines may cause side effects, such as nausea, vomiting, headaches and hot flushes.

Speak to your doctor for more information about the possible side effects of specific medicines.

Medicine that stimulates the ovaries is not recommended for women with unexplained infertility because it has not been found to increase their chances of getting pregnant.

**Surgical procedures**

There are several types of surgical procedures that may be used to investigate fertility problems and help with fertility.

**Fallopian tube surgery**
If your fallopian tubes have become blocked or scarred, you may need surgery to repair them.

Surgery can be used to break up the scar tissue in your fallopian tubes, making it easier for eggs to pass through them.

The success of surgery will depend on the extent of the damage to your fallopian tubes.

Possible complications from tubal surgery include an ectopic pregnancy, which is when the fertilised egg implants outside the womb.

**Endometriosis, fibroids and PCOS:**
Endometriosis is a condition where tissue, similar to the lining of the womb, grows in other places outside the womb.

Laparoscopic surgery is often used to treat endometriosis by destroying or removing fluid-filled sacs called cysts.

It may also be used to remove submucosal fibroids, which are small growths in the womb.

If you have polycystic ovary syndrome (PCOS), a minor surgical procedure called laparoscopic ovarian drilling can be used if ovulation medicine has not worked.

This involves using either heat or a laser to destroy part of the ovary.

**Correcting an epididymal blockage and surgery to retrieve sperm:**
The epididymis is a coil-like structure in the testicles that helps store and transport sperm.

Sometimes the epididymis becomes blocked, preventing sperm from being ejaculated normally. If this is causing infertility, surgery can be used to correct the blockage.

Surgical extraction of sperm may be an option if you:

- Have an obstruction that prevents the release of sperm
- Were born without the tube that drains the sperm from the testicle (vas deferens)

- Have had a vasectomy or a failed vasectomy reversal

Surgical extraction is usually done under local anaesthetic, but might be done under general anaesthetic depending on which type of procedure you have. It will usually be done as an outpatient procedure.

You'll be advised on the same day about the quality of the tissue or sperm collected.

Any sperm will be frozen and placed in storage for use at a later stage.

**Assisted conception**

Intrauterine insemination (IUI)
Intrauterine insemination (IUI), also known as artificial insemination, involves inserting sperm into the womb via a thin plastic tube passed through the cervix.

Sperm is first collected and washed in a fluid. The best quality specimens (the fastest moving) are selected.

**In vitro fertilisation (IVF):**

In vitro fertilisation (IVF), is when an egg is fertilised outside the body. Fertility medicine is taken to encourage the ovaries to produce more eggs than usual.

Eggs are removed from the ovaries and fertilised with sperm in a laboratory. A fertilised egg (embryo) is then returned to the womb to grow and develop.

**Egg and sperm donation:**

If you or your partner has an infertility problem, you may be able to receive eggs or sperm from a donor to help you conceive. Treatment with donor eggs is usually done using IVF.

Anyone who registered to donate eggs or sperm after 1 April 2005 can no longer remain anonymous and must provide information about their identity.

This is because a child born as a result of donated eggs or sperm is legally entitled to find out the identity of the donor when they become an adult (at age 18).

**Adhesions and ovarian cysts**

Some women will develop:

- Adhesions – "sticky" areas of endometriosis tissue that can join organs together
- Ovarian cysts – fluid-filled cysts in the ovaries that can sometimes become very large and painful

These can both occur if the endometriosis tissue is on or near the ovaries.

They can be treated with surgery, but may come back in the future if the endometriosis returns.

**Treatment**

In most cases, ovarian cysts disappear in a few months without the need for treatment.

Whether treatment is needed will depend on:

- Its size and appearance
- Whether you have any symptoms
- Whether you've had the menopause – if you are postmenopausal there is a slightly higher risk of ovarian cancer

## Watchful waiting

In most cases, a policy of "watchful waiting" is recommended.

This means you will not receive immediate treatment, but you may have an ultrasound scan a few weeks or months later to check if the cyst has gone.

If you have been through the menopause you may be advised to have ultrasound scans and blood tests every 4 months for a year, as you will have a slightly higher risk of ovarian cancer.

If the scans show that the cyst has disappeared, further tests and treatment are not usually necessary. Surgery may be recommended if the cyst is still there.

## Surgery

Large or persistent ovarian cysts, or cysts that are causing symptoms, usually need to be surgically removed.

Surgery is also normally recommended if there are concerns that the cyst could be cancerous or could become cancerous.

There are 2 types of surgery used to remove ovarian cysts:

- A laparoscopy
- A laparotomy

These are usually carried out under general anaesthetic.


**Laparoscopy**

Most cysts can be removed using laparoscopy. This is a type of keyhole surgery where small cuts are made in your tummy and gas is blown into the pelvis to allow the surgeon to access your ovaries.

A laparoscope (a small, tube-shaped microscope with a light on the end) is passed into your abdomen so the surgeon can see your internal organs. The surgeon then removes the cyst through the small cuts in your skin.

After the cyst has been removed, the cuts will be closed using dissolvable stitches.

A laparoscopy is preferred because it causes less pain and has a quicker recovery time. Most people are able to go home on the same day or the following day.

**Laparotomy**
If your cyst is particularly large, or there's a chance it could be cancerous, a laparotomy may be recommended.

During a laparotomy, a single, larger cut is made in your tummy to give the surgeon better access to the cyst.

The whole cyst and ovary may be removed and sent to a laboratory to check whether it's cancerous. Stitches or staples will be used to close the incision.

You may need to stay in hospital for a few days after the procedure.

**After surgery**
The time it takes to recover from surgery is different for everyone. After the ovarian cyst has been removed, you'll feel pain in your tummy, although this should improve in a few days.

After a laparoscopy or a laparotomy, it may take as long as 12 weeks before you can resume normal activities.

If the cyst is sent off for testing, the results should come back in a few weeks and your consultant will discuss with you whether you need any further treatment.

Contact a GP if you notice the following symptoms during your recovery:

- Heavy bleeding
- Severe pain or swelling in your abdomen
- A high temperature (fever)
- Dark or smelly vaginal discharge

These symptoms may indicate an infection.

**Your fertility?**
If you have not been through the menopause, your surgeon will try to preserve as much of your reproductive system as they can. It's often possible to just remove the cyst and leave both ovaries intact, which means your fertility should be unaffected.

If 1 of your ovaries needs to be removed, the remaining ovary will still release hormones and eggs as usual. Your fertility should not be affected, although you may find it slightly harder to get pregnant.

Occasionally, it may be necessary to remove both ovaries, even if you have not been through the menopause. This triggers an early menopause and means you no longer produce any eggs.

However, it may still be possible to have a baby by having a donated egg implanted into your womb. This will need to be discussed with specialists at a centre that specialises in assisted reproduction techniques.

If you have been through the menopause, both ovaries may be removed because they no longer produce eggs.

Make sure you discuss your fertility concerns with your surgeon before your operation.

**Surgery complications**

Like all types of surgery, surgery for endometriosis carries a risk of complications.

The more common complications are not usually serious, and can include:

- A wound infection
- Minor bleeding
- Bruising around the wound

Less common, but more serious, risks include:

- Damage to an organ, such as a hole accidentally being made in the womb, bladder or bowel
- Severe bleeding inside the tummy
- A blood clot in the leg DVT (deep vein thrombosis) or lungs (pulmonary embolism)

Before having surgery, talk to your surgeon about the benefits and possible risks involved.

### Bladder and bowel problems

Endometriosis affecting the bladder or bowel can be difficult to treat and may require major surgery.

You may be referred to a specialist endometriosis service if your bladder or bowel is affected.

Surgery for endometriosis that's around or inside the bladder may involve cutting away part of the bladder.

A tube called a urinary catheter may be placed in your bladder to help you pee in the days after surgery.

In a few cases, you may need to pee into a bag attached to a small hole made in your tummy. This is called a urostomy and it's usually temporary.

Treatment for endometriosis that's around or inside the bowel may involve removing a section of bowel.

Some women need to have a temporary colostomy while their bowel heals. This is where the bowel is diverted through a hole in the tummy and waste products are collected in a bag.

## Impact on life

The impact of endometriosis on life can be profound and multifaceted, affecting various aspects including physical health, emotional well-being, relationships, career, and overall quality of life. Here's a breakdown of some key areas:

1. Physical Health: Endometriosis can cause chronic pelvic pain, painful periods (dysmenorrhea), painful intercourse (dyspareunia), digestive issues, fatigue, and other symptoms. These symptoms can significantly impair daily activities and diminish overall physical well-being.

2. Emotional Well-being: Living with chronic pain and unpredictable symptoms can take a toll on mental health. Many individuals with endometriosis experience anxiety, depression, frustration, and feelings of isolation. Coping with the uncertainty of the condition and the challenges of finding effective treatment can exacerbate these emotional struggles.

3. Relationships: Endometriosis can strain relationships with partners, family members, and friends. The condition may impact intimacy and sexual relationships due to pain during intercourse. Additionally, the need for support and

understanding from loved ones can sometimes be met with frustration or misunderstanding, leading to strain in relationships.

4. Career and Education: Endometriosis can interfere with work or school attendance due to pain, fatigue, and other symptoms. Some individuals may need to take time off or make accommodations to manage their condition, which can impact career progression or academic performance. Discrimination or lack of understanding from employers or educators may also present challenges.

5. Fertility and Reproductive Choices: Endometriosis is a leading cause of infertility in women. The condition can affect fertility by causing inflammation, scarring, and structural abnormalities in the reproductive organs. For those who desire children, the diagnosis of endometriosis can bring significant emotional distress and uncertainty about future fertility options.

6. Financial Impact: Managing endometriosis often involves medical expenses, including doctor's visits, diagnostic tests, medications, and possibly surgeries. Additionally, the need for alternative

treatments, such as acupuncture or dietary supplements, may add to the financial burden. For some individuals, the condition may also result in lost income due to time off work or reduced productivity.

Overall, the impact of endometriosis on life is complex and can vary greatly from person to person. It requires a comprehensive approach to management that addresses both the physical and emotional aspects of the condition, while also providing support and understanding from healthcare providers, loved ones, and the broader community.

**Why is my fertility threatened?**
Endometriosis can threaten fertility through various mechanisms, affecting both the structure and function of the reproductive organs, as well as disrupting the hormonal balance necessary for conception. Here's a detailed explanation:

1. Inflammation and Scarring: Endometriosis involves the growth of tissue similar to the lining of the uterus (endometrium) outside of the uterus, typically on the ovaries, fallopian tubes, and other

pelvic organs. This abnormal tissue growth can lead to inflammation and the formation of adhesions or scar tissue in the pelvic cavity. Adhesions can distort the anatomy of the reproductive organs and interfere with the normal function of the fallopian tubes, which are essential for transporting eggs from the ovaries to the uterus.

2. Ovarian Dysfunction: Endometriosis can affect ovarian function and the quality of eggs produced. Inflammation and scarring on the ovaries can impair follicle development and disrupt ovulation, leading to irregular menstrual cycles or anovulation (lack of ovulation). Additionally, endometriomas, which are cysts filled with old blood from endometrial tissue, can develop on the ovaries, further compromising ovarian function and egg quality.

3. Implantation Issues: Endometriosis can create a hostile environment within the pelvic cavity, making it difficult for a fertilized egg (embryo) to implant and establish a pregnancy. Inflammation and scarring in the endometrial lining may impair its ability to support embryo implantation, increasing the risk of implantation failure and early pregnancy loss (miscarriage).

4. Hormonal Imbalance: Endometriosis is associated with hormonal imbalances, particularly elevated levels of estrogen relative to progesterone. This hormonal imbalance can disrupt the delicate interplay of hormones necessary for ovulation, implantation, and maintenance of pregnancy. Additionally, excess estrogen may promote the growth of endometrial tissue outside the uterus, exacerbating the symptoms of endometriosis and further compromising fertility.

5. Treatment Effects: Some treatments for endometriosis, such as surgery to remove endometrial implants or ovarian cysts, may inadvertently damage healthy ovarian tissue or compromise ovarian reserve (the quantity and quality of eggs remaining in the ovaries). In severe cases, where fertility preservation is a concern, surgical interventions may result in the removal of reproductive organs, such as the ovaries or uterus, which can permanently impact fertility.

Overall, the complex interplay of inflammation, scarring, hormonal imbalances, and treatment effects associated with endometriosis can pose significant challenges to fertility. However, it's important to note that not all individuals with endometriosis will experience infertility, and there are various fertility treatments and interventions available to help individuals with endometriosis achieve pregnancy.

# Chapter 2

# Holistic approaches

In the journey of managing endometriosis, a holistic approach to healing recognizes the interconnectedness of mind, body, and spirit in achieving overall well-being. This chapter delves into the fundamental principles of holistic health and explores how adopting a comprehensive approach to care can empower individuals to address the root causes of endometriosis symptoms while promoting long-term healing and vitality.

Holistic health encompasses a broad spectrum of practices and philosophies that prioritize the integration of physical, emotional, and spiritual aspects of health. At its core, holistic healing recognizes that the body possesses innate healing abilities and strives to support these natural processes through a combination of lifestyle interventions, complementary therapies, and mind-body practices.

Central to the holistic approach is the recognition of the mind-body connection and its profound influence on health outcomes. Research has shown that stress, emotions, and psychological factors can impact the severity of endometriosis symptoms and contribute to disease progression. Therefore, strategies for stress management, emotional resilience, and mindfulness play a pivotal role in holistic healing. Techniques such as meditation, yoga, deep breathing exercises, and guided imagery are explored as powerful tools for reducing stress, promoting relaxation, and enhancing overall well-being.

In addition to addressing the emotional aspects of health, a holistic approach to healing also emphasizes the importance of nutrition and lifestyle factors in managing endometriosis. Dietary interventions that focus on reducing inflammation, supporting hormonal balance, and promoting gut health are discussed as key components of a holistic treatment plan. By incorporating anti-inflammatory foods, nourishing nutrients, and gut-healing practices into their diet, individuals with endometriosis can optimize their body's ability to heal and thrive.

Furthermore, holistic healing extends beyond the individual to encompass their environment and social support network. Cultivating supportive relationships, creating a healing environment at home, and fostering a sense of community are integral aspects of holistic care that contribute to overall wellness.

By embracing a holistic approach to healing, individuals with endometriosis can cultivate a sense of empowerment, resilience, and self-care that transcends the limitations of conventional medicine. This chapter serves as a guidepost for navigating the complexities of endometriosis with a comprehensive toolkit for holistic well-being.

## Holistic Health Principles

Holistic health principles embody a comprehensive approach to well-being that integrates the physical, mental, emotional, and spiritual aspects of health. It emphasizes the interconnectedness of these dimensions and recognizes that true health is achieved through balance and harmony within the whole person and their environment. Here's an exhaustive exploration of holistic health principles:

1. Wholeness: Holistic health views the individual as a whole entity, rather than focusing solely on isolated symptoms or body parts. It acknowledges that the mind, body, emotions, and spirit are interconnected and interdependent, and that each aspect influences the overall health and well-being of the individual.

2. Balance: Balance is central to holistic health, emphasizing the importance of equilibrium and harmony within the body and mind. It recognizes that imbalances in one aspect of health can impact other areas, leading to physical symptoms, emotional distress, or spiritual unrest. Achieving balance involves addressing underlying root causes and restoring equilibrium through various interventions.

3. Prevention: Holistic health prioritizes prevention as a proactive approach to maintaining health and preventing disease. It emphasizes lifestyle factors such as nutrition, exercise, stress management, and adequate rest as essential components of disease prevention. By promoting healthy habits and

supporting the body's natural healing mechanisms, holistic health aims to prevent illness before it occurs.

4. Individuality: Holistic health recognizes that each person is unique and that health interventions should be tailored to individual needs, preferences, and circumstances. It acknowledges the importance of personalized care and respects the diversity of human experiences, including cultural, social, and environmental factors that influence health outcomes.

5. Self-Healing: Holistic health believes in the innate healing abilities of the body and mind. It emphasizes the body's natural capacity to heal itself when provided with the right conditions and support. By addressing underlying imbalances and removing obstacles to healing, holistic approaches aim to facilitate the body's self-healing mechanisms and promote optimal health.

6. Mind-Body Connection: Holistic health recognizes the powerful interrelationship between the mind and body and the influence of mental and emotional states on physical health. It acknowledges that emotional stress, trauma, and negative thought

patterns can manifest as physical symptoms or contribute to the development of disease. Therefore, holistic approaches often incorporate mind-body practices such as meditation, yoga, and mindfulness to promote emotional well-being and support physical health.

7. Interconnectedness: Holistic health acknowledges the interconnectedness of individuals with their environment, including social, cultural, and ecological factors. It recognizes that health is influenced by external factors such as social support, environmental toxins, and socioeconomic conditions. Therefore, holistic approaches may address broader systemic issues that impact health outcomes and advocate for environmental and social justice.

By embracing these holistic health principles, individuals can cultivate a deeper understanding of their health and well-being, empowering them to take an active role in their own healing journey and promoting holistic wellness for themselves and their communities.

# Mind-Body Connection

The mind-body connection refers to the intricate relationship between mental and emotional processes and physical health outcomes. It acknowledges that thoughts, emotions, beliefs, and attitudes can influence physiological functioning, immune responses, and overall well-being. Here's a comprehensive exploration of the mind-body connection:

1. Biological Pathways: The mind and body are interconnected through a complex network of biological pathways, including the nervous system, endocrine system, and immune system. For example, stress triggers the release of stress hormones such as cortisol and adrenaline, which can affect heart rate, blood pressure, and immune function. Chronic stress has been linked to a wide range of health conditions, including cardiovascular disease, autoimmune disorders, and gastrointestinal disorders.

2. Emotional Impact on Health: Emotions play a significant role in shaping health outcomes. Positive emotions such as joy, gratitude, and love have been associated with improved immune function,

cardiovascular health, and longevity. Conversely, negative emotions such as anger, fear, and sadness can contribute to inflammation, oxidative stress, and impaired immune function, increasing the risk of chronic diseases and health problems.

3. Psychosomatic Effects: Psychosomatic disorders are conditions in which psychological factors contribute to physical symptoms or illness. Examples include tension headaches, irritable bowel syndrome, and chronic pain syndromes. These conditions illustrate how psychological stressors, such as unresolved trauma, emotional conflicts, or chronic stress, can manifest as physical symptoms in the body.

4. Placebo and Nocebo Effects: The placebo effect refers to the phenomenon where individuals experience improvements in symptoms or health outcomes after receiving a placebo treatment (a sham or inert substance) due to the belief that it will be beneficial. Conversely, the nocebo effect occurs when negative expectations or beliefs lead to the worsening of symptoms or the development of side effects, even when receiving an inactive treatment. These effects highlight the power of the mind in influencing health outcomes.

5. Mind-Body Practices: Mind-body practices encompass a wide range of techniques and interventions that promote the integration of mental, emotional, and physical aspects of health. Examples include meditation, yoga, tai chi, biofeedback, guided imagery, and relaxation techniques. These practices have been shown to reduce stress, promote relaxation, enhance emotional well-being, and improve physical health outcomes.

6. Mindfulness: Mindfulness involves cultivating present moment awareness and non-judgmental acceptance of one's thoughts, feelings, and sensations. Mindfulness practices have been associated with reductions in stress, anxiety, depression, and chronic pain, as well as improvements in immune function, cardiovascular health, and overall quality of life. By fostering greater self-awareness and emotional regulation, mindfulness enhances the mind-body connection and promotes holistic well-being.

Overall, the mind-body connection underscores the inseparable link between mental and physical health and highlights the importance of addressing psychological factors in promoting overall well-being. By cultivating awareness of this connection and incorporating mind-body practices into daily life, individuals can empower themselves to optimize their health and vitality.

## Importance of Stress Management

Stress management is crucial for maintaining overall health and well-being, as chronic stress can have profound effects on both the mind and body. Here's an exploration of the importance of stress management:

1. Physical Health: Chronic stress can take a toll on physical health, contributing to a wide range of health problems including cardiovascular disease, hypertension, diabetes, obesity, gastrointestinal disorders, and immune dysfunction. Prolonged activation of the body's stress response system, including the release of stress hormones such as cortisol and adrenaline, can lead to inflammation, oxidative stress, and dysregulation of physiological processes. By managing stress effectively, individuals can reduce their risk of developing

stress-related illnesses and promote better physical health outcomes.

2. Mental Health: Stress has a significant impact on mental health, contributing to anxiety disorders, depression, insomnia, and other mood disorders. Chronic stress can exacerbate existing mental health conditions and impair cognitive function, memory, and concentration. Effective stress management techniques such as mindfulness, relaxation, and cognitive-behavioral strategies can help alleviate symptoms of anxiety and depression, improve mood, and enhance overall psychological well-being.

3. Immune Function: Prolonged stress has been shown to suppress immune function, making individuals more susceptible to infections, autoimmune disorders, and chronic inflammatory conditions. Stress hormones such as cortisol can inhibit the activity of immune cells, impairing the body's ability to fight off pathogens and heal from injury or illness. By managing stress and reducing its impact on the immune system, individuals can support their body's natural defense mechanisms and enhance resilience to disease.

4. Quality of Life: Chronic stress can significantly diminish quality of life, affecting relationships, work performance, and daily functioning. It can lead to burnout, fatigue, irritability, and feelings of overwhelm. By learning to effectively manage stress, individuals can improve their coping skills, enhance resilience, and experience greater overall satisfaction and fulfillment in life.

5. Longevity: Chronic stress has been linked to accelerated aging and a shortened lifespan. By reducing stress and its impact on physical and mental health, individuals can potentially increase their longevity and enjoy a higher quality of life in their later years.

In summary, stress management is essential for promoting optimal health and well-being. By incorporating stress reduction techniques into daily life, individuals can protect themselves from the harmful effects of chronic stress, enhance resilience, and cultivate a greater sense of balance, peace, and vitality.

## Can endometriosis be cured without surgery?

There are many ways to treat endometriosis, but surgery is often the first option. So is because surgery can remove the growths caused by endometriosis, which can help relieve symptoms. Other treatments include hormone therapy and birth control pills. Some women also find relief through alternative therapies, such as acupuncture or herbal supplements.

There are several ways to reduce the severity of endometriosis without surgery. Some people may choose to take medication to help relieve their symptoms, while others may opt for a more natural approach.

Here are some of the most common ways to cure endometriosis without surgery:

1. Taking medication: There are several medications available to help relieve the symptoms of endometriosis. Some people may find relief by taking over-the-counter painkillers, while others may need to take prescription medication to get relief.

2. Changing your diet: Some people find that changing their diet can help relieve the symptoms of endometriosis. For example, eating a healthy diet

high in fruits and vegetables can help improve your overall health and may help reduce the symptoms of endometriosis.

3. Exercise: Exercise can also help reduce the symptoms of endometriosis. Exercising regularly can help improve your overall health and may help reduce the amount of pain you experience from endometriosis.

4. Using natural remedies: Several natural remedies can help reduce the symptoms of endometriosis. Some people may find relief by using supplements such as ginger or turmeric, while others may find relief by using essential oils such as lavender oil or frankincense oil.

There are many ways to reduce the symptoms of endometriosis without surgery. However, there is no cure for endometriosis. The disease can come back after surgery and often reoccurs within five years.

So, if you are not comfortable with the idea of surgery or have already had surgery and it has not relieved your symptoms, there are other options available to you. If you are experiencing pain and discomfort from endometriosis, it is important to consult with your doctor to find the best treatment.

# Chapter 3

# Natural remedies and supplements

## Home remedies

**1. Heat:**
If your symptoms are acting up and you need relief, heat may help. Heat can relax the pelvic muscles, which can reduce cramping and pain. You can use warm baths, hot water bottles, or heating pads to help treat cramping.

**2. OTC anti-inflammatory drugs:**
Over-the-counter (OTC) nonsteroidal anti-inflammatory drugs (NSAIDs) may offer relief from mild pain caused by endometriosis. These drugs include ibuprofen and naproxen.

It's best to talk with your doctor before taking NSAIDs if you're taking other medications or if you have a history of stomach ulcers.

**3. Bromelain:**
Bromelain is an enzyme found in pineapples that can also be taken as a supplement. Some research

has found that bromelain in combination with the supplement N-acetyl cysteine and the antioxidant alpha lipoic acid significantly reduced pelvic pain from endometriosis.

If you choose to try bromelain supplements, it's important to first check with your doctor as it may interact with some medications.

4. Turmeric:
Turmeric has strong anti-inflammatory properties that may benefit people experiencing endometriosis symptoms.

Some research has found that curcumin, a compound in turmeric, may reduce endometriosis pain. It's still unclear exactly how curcumin achieves this result, but it may reduce inflammation and inhibit the development of endometriosis.

You can take turmeric capsules or you can make turmeric tea using turmeric root or tea bags. Remember to talk with your doctor before taking turmeric or other new supplements.

5. Anti-inflammatory foods

More studies are needed on diet's effects on endometriosis, but some researchTrusted Source indicates that an anti-inflammatory diet may help reduce pain. This won't offer fast symptom relief, but it could help manage the endometriosis long-term.

By avoiding foods that cause inflammation and increasing foods with anti-inflammatory properties in your diet, you may be able to reduce symptoms in the future.

Inflammatory foods to eat less of include:

- Dairy
- Red meat
- Fried foods

Foods to increase include:

- Green tea
- Fatty fish
- Green leafy vegetables
- Berries
- Cherries
- Walnuts
- Olive oil

- Spices

6. Massage:
Some research indicates that massage may help with pain management for people with endometriosis. Another small study found that osteopathy, which involves physical manipulation similar to massage, improved symptoms of endometriosis.

More studies need to be done on the effectiveness of massage for endometriosis. Still, it's a straightforward technique you can try at home to see if it reduces your endometriosis pain.

7. Ginger tea:
Some people with endometriosis experience nausea as a result of the condition. Ginger tea is an established home remedy for treating nausea, and research has consistently shown that it's both safe and effective.

You can purchase ginger tea packets at many supermarkets and grocery stores. When you're experiencing nausea, add one to a cup of boiling water, let it steep, and drink.

8. Yoga:
Yoga is an ancient practice that combines meditation and physical postures. It's often used for stress relief, but may also improve endometriosis symptoms.

A very small study of 15 women with endometriosis found that practicing yoga twice a week for 8 weeks helped reduce pelvic pain. A 2018 research review also indicated that while evidence was inconclusive for the benefits of yoga, it may have the potential to improve endometriosis symptoms.

You can learn yoga poses online or try taking a class in your community.

## Which Herbs Help Endometriosis Symptoms?

Endometriosis is a disorder that affects the reproductive system. It causes endometrium-like tissue to grow outside of the uterus in areas like the ovaries, abdomen, and bowel.

Endometriosis can spread outside the pelvic area, but it typically occurs on the:

- Outer surface of the uterus
- Ovaries
- Fallopian tubes
- Tissues that hold the uterus in place

## Endometriosis herb and spice remedies

Advocates of natural healing suggest herbal remedies may help treat the symptoms of endometriosis. Some of their claims are backed by clinical research.

**Curcumin**
Curcumin is the primary active ingredient in turmeric.

It's known for having anti-inflammatory properties, which was confirmed in a 2009 review.

A 2013 study suggested that curcumin may help with endometriosis by reducing estradiol production. A 2015 study suggested curcumin may suppress tissue migration of the lining of the uterus.

Additionally, a 2018 review discussed the anti-inflammatory, antioxidant, and other mechanisms that might reduce symptoms of endometriosis.

## Chamomile

According to a 2014 review, chamomile can reduce the symptoms of premenstrual syndrome. Some natural healers suggest drinking chamomile tea can help with endometriosis symptoms.

A 2018 study showed that chrysin, a compound found in chamomile, suppressed the growth of endometrial cells.

## Peppermint

According to a 2006 review, peppermint has antioxidant properties. A 2013 studyTrusted Source concluded that antioxidant supplements can reduce pelvic pain from endometriosis.

A 2016 study showed that peppermint can reduce the severity of pain from menstrual cramps.

## Lavender

A 2012 study indicated that women reduced menstrual cramps by using diluted lavender oil in aromatherapy massage. Lavender might help with severe menstrual cramps triggered by endometriosis.

Another 2015 study found lavender oil massage was effective in decreasing pain in periods.

**Ginger**
A 2014 study and a 2016 review both found that ginger can reduce menstruation-related pain. This suggests ginger could have a similar effect on pain associated with endometriosis.

**Cinnamon, clove, rose, and lavender**
A 2013 study tested a mixture of cinnamon, clove, rose, and lavender essential oils in a base of almond oil. The study found it was effective for reducing menstrual pain and bleeding when used in aromatherapy massage.

Proponents of natural healing suggest that the same mixture may have similar results for endometriosis. More studies are needed on blends of herbs and essential oils, but there's little risk if they're used correctly.

**Ashwagandha**

A 2014 review found that clinically significant reductions in stress resulted from treatment with the herb ashwagandha.

A 2006 study found that women with advanced endometriosis had significantly higher levels of cortisol, a hormone involved in stress response.

These studies indicate a potential role for ashwagandha in stress reduction for women with endometriosis.
Symptoms can vary from mild irritation to severe pelvic pain. There's no cure for the condition, but treatment can help manage the symptoms.

Traditional treatments include pain medication, hormone therapy, and medication that blocks the production of estrogen. If you're looking into alternative treatments, you may have heard that certain herbs may be an effective treatment.

# Chapter 4

# Healing recipe

A healing diet is a nutritional approach designed to support the body's natural healing processes, promote optimal health, and alleviate symptoms of illness or disease. It emphasizes whole, nutrient-dense foods that provide essential vitamins, minerals, antioxidants, and phytonutrients necessary for cellular repair, immune function, and overall well-being.

## Breakfast recipes

**Chicken Curry with vegetable**

Ingredients:
- 2 tablespoons oil (such as vegetable or coconut oil)
- 1 onion, chopped
- 3 cloves garlic, minced
- 1 tablespoon ginger, minced
- 1 red bell pepper, sliced

- 1 green bell pepper, sliced
- 2 carrots, sliced
- 1 cup green beans, trimmed and cut into 1-inch pieces
- 1 pound boneless, skinless chicken breasts, cut into bite-sized pieces
- 2 tablespoons curry powder
- 1 teaspoon turmeric powder
- 1 teaspoon ground cumin
- 1 teaspoon ground coriander
- 1/2 teaspoon cayenne pepper (adjust to taste)
- 1 can (14 ounces) coconut milk
- 1 cup chicken broth
- Salt and pepper, to taste
- Fresh cilantro, for garnish
- Cooked rice, for serving

Instructions:

1. Heat the oil in a large skillet or pot over medium heat. Add the chopped onion and cook until softened, about 5 minutes.

2. Add the minced garlic and ginger to the skillet and cook for another 1-2 minutes, until fragrant.

3. Add the sliced red bell pepper, green bell pepper, carrots, and green beans to the skillet. Cook for 5-7 minutes, until the vegetables begin to soften.

4. Push the vegetables to one side of the skillet and add the chicken pieces to the other side. Cook the chicken until browned on all sides, about 5-7 minutes.

5. Stir in the curry powder, turmeric powder, ground cumin, ground coriander, and cayenne pepper. Cook for 1-2 minutes, until the spices are fragrant.

6. Pour in the coconut milk and chicken broth, stirring to combine. Bring the mixture to a simmer.

7. Reduce the heat to low and cover the skillet. Let the curry simmer for 20-25 minutes, stirring occasionally, until the chicken is cooked through and the vegetables are tender.

8. Season the curry with salt and pepper, to taste.

9. Serve the chicken curry with cooked rice and garnish with fresh cilantro.

10. Enjoy your delicious Chicken Curry with Vegetables!

Feel free to adjust the spice levels and vegetables according to your preferences. This flavorful and comforting dish is perfect for a cozy meal at home.

## Vegan Banana Oat Pancake

Ingredients:
- 1 ripe banana

- 1 cup rolled oats
- 1/2 cup non-dairy milk (such as almond milk, soy milk, or coconut milk)
- 1 tablespoon maple syrup or agave syrup (optional, for sweetness)
- 1 teaspoon baking powder
- 1/2 teaspoon vanilla extract
- 1/4 teaspoon ground cinnamon (optional)
- Pinch of salt
- Oil or vegan butter, for cooking

Instructions:

1. In a blender or food processor, combine the ripe banana, rolled oats, non-dairy milk, maple syrup (if using), baking powder, vanilla extract, ground cinnamon (if using), and a pinch of salt. Blend until smooth and well combined. If the batter is too thick, you can add a little more non-dairy milk to reach your desired consistency.

2. Let the pancake batter rest for about 5 minutes to allow the oats to absorb the liquid and thicken slightly.

3. Heat a non-stick skillet or griddle over medium heat. Lightly grease the skillet with oil or vegan butter.

4. Pour a small amount of pancake batter onto the skillet, using about 1/4 cup for each pancake. Use

the back of a spoon or a spatula to spread the batter into a round shape.
5. Cook the pancakes for 2-3 minutes, or until bubbles begin to form on the surface and the edges look set.
6. Carefully flip the pancakes and cook for an additional 2-3 minutes on the other side, or until golden brown and cooked through.
7. Repeat with the remaining batter, adding more oil or vegan butter to the skillet as needed.
8. Serve the vegan banana oat pancakes warm, topped with sliced bananas, fresh berries, a drizzle of maple syrup, or your favorite toppings.
9. Enjoy your delicious and nutritious Vegan Banana Oat Pancakes!

These pancakes are not only vegan-friendly but also gluten-free and packed with fiber and nutrients from the bananas and oats. They make a wholesome and satisfying breakfast or brunch option for anyone looking for a healthier alternative to traditional pancakes.

**Superfood Cereals**

Superfood cereals are nutrient-dense breakfast options packed with a variety of health-promoting ingredients. They typically include a combination of whole grains, seeds, nuts, and dried fruits, along with superfoods known for their exceptional nutritional benefits. Here's a recipe for a homemade superfood cereal:

Ingredients:
- 2 cups rolled oats
- 1/2 cup quinoa, rinsed
- 1/2 cup raw almonds, chopped
- 1/2 cup raw walnuts, chopped
- 1/4 cup pumpkin seeds
- 1/4 cup sunflower seeds
- 1/4 cup chia seeds
- 1/4 cup flaxseeds
- 1/4 cup dried goji berries
- 1/4 cup dried cranberries
- 1/4 cup dried blueberries
- 1/4 cup dried apricots, chopped
- 1/4 cup dried coconut flakes
- 2 tablespoons maple syrup or honey (optional, for sweetness)
- 1 tablespoon coconut oil, melted
- 1 teaspoon ground cinnamon
- Pinch of salt

Instructions:

1. Preheat your oven to 300°F (150°C) and line a baking sheet with parchment paper.

2. In a large mixing bowl, combine the rolled oats, quinoa, chopped almonds, chopped walnuts, pumpkin seeds, sunflower seeds, chia seeds, flaxseeds, dried goji berries, dried cranberries, dried blueberries, chopped apricots, and dried coconut flakes. Mix well to combine.

3. In a small bowl, whisk together the maple syrup or honey (if using), melted coconut oil, ground cinnamon, and a pinch of salt.

4. Pour the wet ingredients over the dry ingredients and toss until everything is evenly coated.

5. Spread the mixture evenly onto the prepared baking sheet in a single layer.

6. Bake in the preheated oven for 25-30 minutes, stirring occasionally, until the cereal is golden brown and toasted.

7. Remove from the oven and let cool completely on the baking sheet.

8. Once cooled, transfer the superfood cereal to an airtight container for storage.

9. Serve with your favorite non-dairy milk or yogurt, fresh fruit, and a drizzle of honey or maple syrup, if desired.

10. Enjoy your homemade superfood cereal as a nutritious and satisfying breakfast or snack option!

Feel free to customize this recipe by adding or substituting different nuts, seeds, and dried fruits based on your preferences and dietary needs. This superfood cereal is rich in fiber, protein, healthy fats, vitamins, and antioxidants, making it a nourishing and energizing way to start your day.

## Anti-inflammatory blueberry

Blueberries are considered a superfood due to their high antioxidant content, particularly anthocyanins, which give them their vibrant color and anti-inflammatory properties. Here's a recipe for an anti-inflammatory blueberry smoothie:

Ingredients:
- 1 cup fresh or frozen blueberries
- 1/2 cup spinach or kale
- 1/2 cup Greek yogurt or dairy-free yogurt alternative
- 1 tablespoon chia seeds
- 1 tablespoon hemp seeds
- 1/2 inch fresh ginger, peeled and grated
- 1 teaspoon turmeric powder
- 1 teaspoon cinnamon

- 1 tablespoon honey or maple syrup (optional, for sweetness)
- 1 cup unsweetened almond milk or coconut water

Instructions:
1. Place all ingredients in a blender.
2. Blend on high until smooth and creamy.
3. Taste and adjust sweetness, if necessary, by adding honey or maple syrup.
4. Pour into glasses and serve immediately.
5. Enjoy your refreshing and anti-inflammatory blueberry smoothie!

This smoothie is not only delicious but also packed with nutrients that support inflammation reduction and overall health. Blueberries provide antioxidants, while spinach or kale offer additional vitamins and minerals. Chia seeds and hemp seeds add fiber, protein, and omega-3 fatty acids, while ginger and turmeric provide anti-inflammatory benefits. Cinnamon adds warmth and flavor, making this smoothie a nutritious and tasty way to start your day or refuel after a workout.

# Lunch recipes

## Roasted Vegetables and Hummus Wrap

Roasted vegetables and hummus make for a delicious and satisfying wrap that's packed with flavor and nutrients. Here's a recipe for a Roasted Vegetables and Hummus Wrap:

Ingredients:
- 1 large whole wheat or spinach tortilla wrap
- 1/4 cup hummus (store-bought or homemade)
- 1 cup mixed roasted vegetables (such as bell peppers, zucchini, eggplant, cherry tomatoes, red onion)
- Handful of fresh spinach or arugula leaves
- 1/4 cup crumbled feta cheese or dairy-free cheese alternative (optional)
- 1 tablespoon chopped fresh herbs (such as parsley, basil, or cilantro)
- Salt and pepper, to taste
- Olive oil, for roasting vegetables

Instructions:
1. Preheat your oven to 400°F (200°C).

2. Place the mixed vegetables on a baking sheet lined with parchment paper. Drizzle with olive oil and season with salt and pepper to taste. Toss to coat evenly.

3. Roast the vegetables in the preheated oven for 20-25 minutes, or until tender and slightly caramelized. Remove from the oven and let cool slightly.

4. Warm the tortilla wrap in a dry skillet over medium heat for 30 seconds on each side, or until soft and pliable.

5. Spread the hummus evenly over the center of the tortilla wrap, leaving a border around the edges.

6. Layer the roasted vegetables on top of the hummus, followed by the fresh spinach or arugula leaves.

7. If using, sprinkle crumbled feta cheese or dairy-free cheese alternative over the vegetables.

8. Sprinkle chopped fresh herbs over the top for added flavor.

9. Fold the sides of the tortilla wrap over the filling, then roll it up tightly from the bottom to enclose the ingredients.

10. Slice the wrap in half diagonally, if desired, and serve immediately.

11. Enjoy your delicious and nutritious Roasted Vegetables and Hummus Wrap!

This wrap is versatile and customizable, so feel free to add or substitute your favorite roasted vegetables, greens, or additional toppings such as avocado slices, olives, or pickled onions. It's perfect for a quick and healthy lunch or dinner option that's both satisfying and full of flavor.

**Lentil and Vegetable Stew**

Lentil and vegetable stew is a hearty and nutritious dish that's perfect for cold weather or anytime you're craving a comforting meal. Here's a recipe to make a delicious Lentil and Vegetable Stew:

Ingredients:
- 1 tablespoon olive oil
- 1 onion, diced
- 3 cloves garlic, minced
- 2 carrots, diced
- 2 celery stalks, diced
- 1 bell pepper, diced (any color)
- 1 cup dried green or brown lentils, rinsed and drained
- 1 can (14 ounces) diced tomatoes
- 4 cups vegetable broth
- 1 teaspoon dried thyme

- 1 teaspoon dried oregano
- 1 teaspoon paprika
- 1/2 teaspoon cumin
- Salt and pepper, to taste
- 2 cups chopped leafy greens (such as kale, spinach, or Swiss chard)
- Fresh parsley, for garnish (optional)

Instructions:
1. Heat the olive oil in a large pot or Dutch oven over medium heat.
2. Add the diced onion and cook until softened, about 5 minutes.
3. Add the minced garlic and cook for an additional 1-2 minutes, until fragrant.
4. Stir in the diced carrots, celery, and bell pepper. Cook for 5-7 minutes, until the vegetables begin to soften.
5. Add the rinsed lentils, diced tomatoes (with their juices), vegetable broth, dried thyme, dried oregano, paprika, and cumin to the pot. Stir to combine.
6. Bring the stew to a boil, then reduce the heat to low and simmer, covered, for 25-30 minutes, or until the lentils are tender.
7. Season the stew with salt and pepper, to taste.
8. Stir in the chopped leafy greens and cook for an additional 5 minutes, until wilted.

9. Taste and adjust seasoning, if necessary.
10. Ladle the lentil and vegetable stew into bowls and garnish with fresh parsley, if desired.
11. Serve hot and enjoy your delicious Lentil and Vegetable Stew!

This stew is versatile, so feel free to customize it with your favorite vegetables, herbs, or spices. It's rich in fiber, protein, vitamins, and minerals, making it a satisfying and nutritious meal option for vegetarians and vegans alike. Serve it with crusty bread or over cooked grains like rice or quinoa for a complete and filling meal.

**Chickpea and sweet potato**

Chickpea and sweet potato stew is a delicious and nutritious dish that's perfect for a cozy meal. Here's a recipe to make Chickpea and Sweet Potato Stew:

Ingredients:
- 1 tablespoon olive oil
- 1 onion, diced
- 3 cloves garlic, minced
- 2 medium sweet potatoes, peeled and diced
- 1 can (15 ounces) chickpeas, rinsed and drained

- 1 can (14 ounces) diced tomatoes
- 4 cups vegetable broth
- 1 teaspoon ground cumin
- 1 teaspoon smoked paprika
- 1/2 teaspoon ground cinnamon
- Salt and pepper, to taste
- 2 cups chopped spinach or kale
- Fresh cilantro, for garnish (optional)
- Cooked rice or quinoa, for serving

Instructions:

1. Heat the olive oil in a large pot or Dutch oven over medium heat.

2. Add the diced onion and cook until softened, about 5 minutes.

3. Add the minced garlic and cook for an additional 1-2 minutes, until fragrant.

4. Stir in the diced sweet potatoes, chickpeas, diced tomatoes (with their juices), vegetable broth, ground cumin, smoked paprika, and ground cinnamon. Stir to combine.

5. Bring the stew to a boil, then reduce the heat to low and simmer, covered, for 20-25 minutes, or until the sweet potatoes are tender.

6. Season the stew with salt and pepper, to taste.

7. Stir in the chopped spinach or kale and cook for an additional 5 minutes, until wilted.

8. Taste and adjust seasoning, if necessary.
9. Ladle the chickpea and sweet potato stew into bowls.
10. Garnish with fresh cilantro, if desired.
11. Serve hot with cooked rice or quinoa on the side.
12. Enjoy your delicious and nutritious Chickpea and Sweet Potato Stew!

This stew is rich in fiber, protein, vitamins, and minerals, making it a satisfying and wholesome meal option. The combination of chickpeas and sweet potatoes provides a hearty texture and sweet flavor, while the warming spices add depth and complexity to the dish. Serve it as a main course for a vegetarian or vegan dinner, or as a side dish alongside grilled chicken or fish.

## Dinner recipes

**Roasted Vegetables and Brown rice Bowl with Tahini Dressing**

Roasted vegetables and brown rice bowl with tahini dressing is a wholesome and flavorful meal that's easy to prepare and packed with nutrients. Here's a

recipe to make Roasted Vegetables and Brown
Rice Bowl with Tahini Dressing:

Ingredients:
For the Roasted Vegetables:
- 2 cups mixed vegetables (such as bell
  peppers, zucchini, eggplant, cherry tomatoes,
  red onion), chopped
- 2 tablespoons olive oil
- 1 teaspoon dried herbs (such as thyme,
  rosemary, or oregano)
- Salt and pepper, to taste

For the Brown Rice:
- 1 cup brown rice, rinsed
- 2 cups water or vegetable broth
- Pinch of salt

For the Tahini Dressing:
- 1/4 cup tahini
- 2 tablespoons lemon juice
- 2 tablespoons water
- 1 clove garlic, minced
- 1 teaspoon maple syrup or honey (optional)
- Salt and pepper, to taste

Optional Toppings:

- Fresh herbs (such as parsley or cilantro), chopped
- Toasted sesame seeds
- Sliced avocado
- Chickpeas or tofu, roasted or grilled

Instructions:
1. Preheat your oven to 400°F (200°C).
2. In a large mixing bowl, toss the chopped mixed vegetables with olive oil, dried herbs, salt, and pepper until well coated.
3. Spread the seasoned vegetables in a single layer on a baking sheet lined with parchment paper.
4. Roast the vegetables in the preheated oven for 20-25 minutes, or until tender and slightly caramelized, stirring halfway through cooking.
5. While the vegetables are roasting, prepare the brown rice. In a medium saucepan, combine the rinsed brown rice, water or vegetable broth, and a pinch of salt. Bring to a boil, then reduce the heat to low, cover, and simmer for 40-45 minutes, or until the rice is tender and the liquid is absorbed. Remove from heat and let stand for 5 minutes before fluffing with a fork.
6. To make the tahini dressing, whisk together the tahini, lemon juice, water, minced garlic, maple syrup or honey (if using), salt, and pepper in a small

bowl until smooth and creamy. Adjust the consistency with more water if necessary.
7. To assemble the bowls, divide the cooked brown rice among serving bowls. Top with the roasted vegetables and any optional toppings of your choice.
8. Drizzle the tahini dressing over the bowls just before serving.
9. Garnish with fresh herbs and toasted sesame seeds, if desired.
10. Serve immediately and enjoy your delicious Roasted Vegetables and Brown Rice Bowl with Tahini Dressing!

This meal is customizable, so feel free to swap out the vegetables or add your favorite protein sources to make it your own. It's a satisfying and nutritious option for lunch or dinner that's sure to please vegans and non-vegans alike.

## Vegan Stuffed Peppers with Quinoa and Black Beans

Vegan stuffed peppers with quinoa and black beans are a nutritious and flavorful dish that's perfect for a wholesome meal. Here's a recipe to make Vegan Stuffed Peppers with Quinoa and Black Beans:

Ingredients:
- 4 large bell peppers, any color
- 1 cup quinoa, rinsed
- 1 can (15 ounces) black beans, drained and rinsed
- 1 cup corn kernels (fresh, frozen, or canned)
- 1 onion, diced
- 2 cloves garlic, minced
- 1 teaspoon ground cumin
- 1 teaspoon chili powder
- 1/2 teaspoon smoked paprika
- Salt and pepper, to taste
- 1 cup tomato sauce or salsa
- 1/2 cup vegan shredded cheese (optional)
- Fresh cilantro, for garnish (optional)
- Lime wedges, for serving (optional)

Instructions:
1. Preheat your oven to 375°F (190°C).
2. Cut the tops off the bell peppers and remove the seeds and membranes. Set aside.
3. In a medium saucepan, bring 2 cups of water to a boil. Add the quinoa, reduce the heat to low, cover, and simmer for 15-20 minutes, or until the quinoa is

cooked and the water is absorbed. Remove from heat and fluff the quinoa with a fork.

4. In a large skillet, heat olive oil over medium heat. Add the diced onion and cook until softened, about 5 minutes.

5. Add the minced garlic, ground cumin, chili powder, smoked paprika, salt, and pepper to the skillet. Cook for an additional 1-2 minutes, until fragrant.

6. Stir in the cooked quinoa, black beans, and corn kernels until well combined. Cook for 2-3 minutes, until heated through.

7. Pour the tomato sauce or salsa into the bottom of a baking dish.

8. Stuff each bell pepper with the quinoa and black bean mixture, pressing down gently to pack the filling.

9. Place the stuffed peppers upright in the baking dish.

10. If using, sprinkle vegan shredded cheese over the top of each stuffed pepper.

11. Cover the baking dish with aluminum foil and bake in the preheated oven for 25-30 minutes, or until the peppers are tender.

12. Remove the foil and bake for an additional 5-10 minutes, or until the cheese is melted and bubbly (if using).

13. Remove from the oven and let cool for a few minutes before serving.
14. Garnish with fresh cilantro and serve with lime wedges on the side, if desired.
15. Enjoy your delicious Vegan Stuffed Peppers with Quinoa and Black Beans!

These stuffed peppers are packed with protein, fiber, vitamins, and minerals, making them a satisfying and nutritious meal option for vegans and non-vegans alike. Serve them as a main course for dinner or as a hearty lunch option. They're also great for meal prep and leftovers can be enjoyed the next day.

**Chickpea Falafels with Pumpkin Hummus**

Chickpea falafels with pumpkin hummus is a flavorful and satisfying dish that's perfect for a vegetarian or vegan meal. Here's a recipe to make Chickpea Falafels with Pumpkin Hummus:

Ingredients for Chickpea Falafels:
- 2 cups cooked chickpeas (or 1 can, drained and rinsed)
- 1/2 cup fresh parsley, chopped

- 1/4 cup fresh cilantro, chopped
- 3 cloves garlic, minced
- 1 small onion, chopped
- 2 tablespoons lemon juice
- 2 teaspoons ground cumin
- 1 teaspoon ground coriander
- 1/2 teaspoon ground paprika
- 1/4 teaspoon cayenne pepper (optional, for heat)
- Salt and pepper, to taste
- 2-3 tablespoons chickpea flour or all-purpose flour
- Olive oil, for frying

Ingredients for Pumpkin Hummus:
- 1 can (15 ounces) chickpeas, drained and rinsed
- 1/2 cup canned pumpkin puree
- 2 tablespoons tahini
- 2 tablespoons lemon juice
- 2 cloves garlic, minced
- 1 teaspoon ground cumin
- 1/2 teaspoon ground paprika
- Salt and pepper, to taste
- Water, as needed

Instructions for Chickpea Falafels:

1. In a food processor, combine the cooked chickpeas, chopped parsley, chopped cilantro, minced garlic, chopped onion, lemon juice, ground cumin, ground coriander, ground paprika, cayenne pepper (if using), salt, and pepper. Pulse until the mixture is well combined but still slightly chunky.
2. Transfer the mixture to a bowl and stir in the chickpea flour or all-purpose flour until the mixture holds together. If the mixture is too wet, add more flour as needed.
3. Shape the mixture into small patties or balls and place them on a baking sheet lined with parchment paper.
4. Heat olive oil in a large skillet over medium heat. Fry the falafels in batches until golden brown and crispy on all sides, about 3-4 minutes per side. Transfer to a plate lined with paper towels to drain excess oil.

Instructions for Pumpkin Hummus:
1. In a food processor, combine the chickpeas, pumpkin puree, tahini, lemon juice, minced garlic, ground cumin, ground paprika, salt, and pepper. Blend until smooth and creamy.
2. If the hummus is too thick, add water, 1 tablespoon at a time, until you reach your desired consistency.

3. Taste and adjust seasoning, if necessary.

To Serve:
1. Serve the chickpea falafels with the pumpkin hummus on the side or spooned over the top.
2. Garnish with additional chopped parsley or cilantro, if desired.
3. Serve as an appetizer, snack, or main course, accompanied by pita bread, fresh vegetables, or a salad.

Enjoy your delicious Chickpea Falafels with Pumpkin Hummus!

# Snacks

## Chia seeds pudding

Chia seed pudding is a delicious and nutritious breakfast or snack option made by soaking chia seeds in a liquid until they expand and become gelatinous. Here's a simple recipe to make chia seed pudding:

Ingredients:
- 1/4 cup chia seeds

- 1 cup almond milk, coconut milk, or any milk of your choice
- 1-2 tablespoons maple syrup, honey, or sweetener of your choice (optional)
- 1/2 teaspoon vanilla extract (optional)
- Fresh fruit, nuts, seeds, or granola for topping (optional)

Instructions:

1. In a mixing bowl or jar, combine the chia seeds, milk, sweetener (if using), and vanilla extract (if using). Stir well to combine.

2. Cover the bowl or jar and refrigerate for at least 2 hours, or overnight, to allow the chia seeds to absorb the liquid and thicken.

3. After the pudding has thickened, give it a good stir to break up any clumps and distribute the seeds evenly.

4. Serve the chia seed pudding in bowls or jars, and top with your favorite fruits, nuts, seeds, or granola for added flavor and texture.

5. Enjoy your delicious and nutritious chia seed pudding!

Chia seed pudding is versatile, so feel free to customize it with different flavors and toppings to suit your taste preferences. It's high in fiber, protein, omega-3 fatty acids, and antioxidants, making it a healthy and satisfying choice for breakfast or snack time. Plus, it's quick and easy to prepare, requiring just a few simple ingredients and minimal effort.

Mixed nuts and Dried Fruits

Mixed nuts and dried fruits make for a delicious and nutritious snack that's perfect for on-the-go or as a mid-day pick-me-up. Here's how you can create your own mix:

Ingredients:
- Assorted nuts (such as almonds, walnuts, cashews, pecans, pistachios)
- Assorted dried fruits (such as raisins, cranberries, apricots, dates, figs, mangoes, apples)

Instructions:
1. Start by selecting your favorite nuts and dried fruits. You can choose a variety of nuts for different textures and flavors, and mix and match your preferred dried fruits for sweetness and chewiness.
2. If your nuts are raw, you can roast them in the oven for added flavor. Spread the nuts in a single

layer on a baking sheet and roast in a preheated oven at 350°F (175°C) for 8-10 minutes, or until fragrant and lightly toasted. Let them cool before mixing with the dried fruits.

3. Once the nuts are cooled, combine them with your chosen dried fruits in a large bowl.

4. Mix well to evenly distribute the nuts and fruits.

5. Store the mixed nuts and dried fruits in an airtight container or resealable bag at room temperature for up to several weeks, or in the refrigerator for longer shelf life.

Enjoy your homemade mixed nuts and dried fruits as a snack on their own, or use them to add flavor and crunch to yogurt, oatmeal, salads, or baked goods. It's a convenient and nutritious snack option that's packed with protein, fiber, healthy fats, vitamins, and minerals to keep you fueled and satisfied throughout the day. Plus, it's customizable to your taste preferences and dietary needs, making it a versatile and delicious choice for anytime snacking.

## Drinks and Dessert

**Ginger Tea**

Ginger tea is a soothing and warming beverage made from fresh ginger root. It's known for its invigorating flavor and potential health benefits, including aiding digestion, reducing inflammation, and relieving nausea. Here's a simple recipe to make ginger tea at home:

Ingredients:
- 1-inch piece of fresh ginger root
- 2 cups water
- Optional: honey, lemon slices, or other natural sweeteners or flavors

Instructions:
1. Peel the ginger root using a spoon or vegetable peeler, then thinly slice it into rounds or grate it using a fine grater.
2. In a small saucepan, bring the water to a boil.
3. Add the sliced or grated ginger to the boiling water.
4. Reduce the heat to low and let the ginger simmer in the water for 10-15 minutes, allowing the flavors to infuse.
5. Remove the saucepan from the heat and let the ginger tea cool slightly.

6. Strain the ginger tea through a fine mesh sieve or cheesecloth to remove the ginger pieces.
7. If desired, sweeten the ginger tea with honey, lemon slices, or other natural sweeteners or flavors to taste.
8. Pour the strained ginger tea into cups and serve hot.
9. Enjoy your homemade ginger tea!

Ginger tea can be enjoyed on its own as a soothing and caffeine-free beverage, or you can customize it with other ingredients like lemon slices or fresh mint leaves for added flavor. It's a comforting drink that's perfect for warming up on chilly days or for relaxing and unwinding in the evening. Plus, it's easy to make and requires just a few simple ingredients. Experiment with different variations to find your favorite way to enjoy ginger tea!

## Aloe Vera Juice

Aloe vera juice is a popular beverage made from the inner gel of the aloe vera plant. It's known for its potential health benefits, including digestive support, hydration, and skin health. Here's a simple recipe to make aloe vera juice at home:

Ingredients:
- 1 large aloe vera leaf (or 2-3 small leaves)
- 1-2 cups water
- Optional: honey, lemon juice, or other natural sweeteners or flavors

Instructions:
1. Wash the aloe vera leaf thoroughly under running water to remove any dirt or debris.
2. Using a sharp knife, carefully slice off the spiky edges of the aloe vera leaf and cut it lengthwise to expose the inner gel.
3. Scoop out the gel from the leaf using a spoon and place it in a blender.
4. Add 1-2 cups of water to the blender, depending on how thick you want your aloe vera juice to be.
5. Blend the mixture on high speed until smooth and well combined.
6. Strain the blended mixture through a fine mesh sieve or cheesecloth to remove any pulp or debris. You can skip this step if you prefer a thicker juice with pulp.
7. If desired, sweeten the aloe vera juice with honey, lemon juice, or other natural sweeteners or flavors to taste.

8. Transfer the strained juice to a clean glass jar or bottle and refrigerate until chilled.
9. Serve the aloe vera juice cold over ice cubes and enjoy!

Aloe vera juice can be consumed on its own as a refreshing beverage or mixed with other juices or smoothies for added nutrition. It's important to note that while aloe vera juice is generally considered safe for consumption, some people may experience digestive discomfort or allergic reactions. If you're new to aloe vera juice, start with a small amount and gradually increase your intake to assess your tolerance. Additionally, consult with your healthcare provider before regularly consuming aloe vera juice, especially if you have any underlying health conditions or are taking medications.

**Turmeric Latte**

Turmeric latte, also known as golden milk, is a warm and comforting beverage made with turmeric and other spices. Here's a simple recipe to make a delicious turmeric latte at home:

Ingredients:

- 1 cup milk of your choice (such as cow's milk, almond milk, coconut milk)
- 1/2 teaspoon ground turmeric
- 1/4 teaspoon ground cinnamon
- 1/8 teaspoon ground ginger
- Pinch of ground black pepper (optional)
- Sweetener of your choice (such as honey, maple syrup, or agave syrup), to taste
- 1/2 teaspoon coconut oil or ghee (optional, for added creaminess)

Instructions:

1. In a small saucepan, heat the milk over medium-low heat until warm but not boiling.

2. Add the ground turmeric, ground cinnamon, ground ginger, and ground black pepper (if using) to the warm milk.

3. Whisk the mixture gently until the spices are well combined and the milk is heated through. Be careful not to let it boil.

4. Remove the saucepan from the heat and stir in your preferred sweetener, adjusting the amount to taste.

5. If desired, add coconut oil or ghee to the latte for added creaminess. Stir until melted and well incorporated.

6. Pour the turmeric latte into a mug and enjoy immediately.

Turmeric latte is known for its vibrant golden color and warming spices, making it a cozy and comforting drink, especially during colder months. Turmeric is also celebrated for its potential health benefits, thanks to its anti-inflammatory and antioxidant properties. Feel free to customize the recipe by adjusting the spices and sweetener to suit your taste preferences. Enjoy your homemade turmeric latte as a soothing and nourishing beverage any time of the day!

# Chapter 5

# Nutrition for endometriosis

Nutrition plays a vital role in managing endometriosis symptoms and promoting overall well-being. A balanced diet focused on whole, nutrient-dense foods can help alleviate inflammation, support hormone balance, and improve overall health.

Incorporate plenty of fruits, vegetables, whole grains, nuts, seeds, and fatty fish into your diet. These foods are rich in antioxidants, fiber, and omega-3 fatty acids, which can help reduce inflammation and support immune function.

Limit intake of processed foods, refined carbohydrates, sugary snacks, and fried foods, as these can exacerbate inflammation and worsen symptoms.

Include plant-based protein sources such as beans, lentils, tofu, and tempeh, which are lower in saturated fat and can help support hormone balance.

Ensure adequate intake of calcium-rich foods like dairy products, fortified plant-based milk alternatives, leafy greens, tofu, almonds, and sesame seeds to support bone health.

Maintain proper hydration by drinking plenty of water throughout the day, as dehydration can worsen symptoms like bloating and constipation.

Consider incorporating herbal teas with anti-inflammatory or calming properties, such as ginger, turmeric, chamomile, or peppermint tea, into your routine.

Consult with a healthcare provider or registered dietitian to develop a personalized nutrition plan tailored to your individual needs and preferences. Remember that while dietary changes can complement medical treatment, they are not a substitute for professional medical advice and care.

**Why food is an aggravating factor for endometriosis?**

Endometriosis is a hormone-dependent condition, meaning nutrition can help treat or manage it. Food significantly influences hormone production and maintenance, immune and inflammatory responses, and smooth muscle contraction.

Additionally, we know that the Western diet has changed hugely over the last few decades with increased consumption of processed foods and refined sugar and decreased consumption of whole foods, fruit, and vegetables. So, food and nutrient intake can significantly impact a hormone-related condition like endometriosis.

## What to eat

To fight inflammation and pain caused by endometriosis, it's best to consume a nutrient-dense, well-balanced diet that's primarily plant-based and full of vitamins and minerals. Add these to your diet:

- fibrous foods, such as fruits, vegetables, legumes, and whole grains
- iron-rich foods, such as dark leafy greens, broccoli, beans, fortified grains, nuts, and seeds

- foods rich in essential fatty acids, such as salmon, sardines, herring, trout, walnuts, chia, and flax seeds
- antioxidant-rich foods found in colorful fruits and vegetables, such as oranges, berries, dark chocolate, spinach, and beets

Make sure you pay attention to how your body acts when you eat certain foods. Keeping a journal of the foods you eat and any symptoms or triggers you have may be helpful.

Consider meeting with a registered dietitian. They can help you plan meals that work best with you and endometriosis, as there's no one-size-fits-all approach.

## What to avoid

Although the exact impact of diet on endometriosis needs further research, evidence suggests that avoiding certain foods can make your condition more manageable.

**Trans fats**

Trans fats or trans-unsaturated fatty acids are found mainly in fried and processed foods, including most fast foods. A 2010 study that considered data from the Nurses Health Study II found that participants with the highest consumption of trans-unsaturated fat were 48% more likely to receive a future endometriosis diagnosis[1].

## Polyunsaturated fats

Omega-6 fatty acid and arachidonic acid are two main polyunsaturated fats, and their impact on endometriosis is well-studied. The two acids eventually metabolize into prostaglandins[2] that cause pain and inflammation. High levels result in inflammation and muscle spasms (cramping).

On the other hand, in one particular study, women with the highest levels of omega-3 fatty acid had a 22% reduction in endometriosis[3].

Research also indicates that omega-3 fatty acids are anti-inflammatory[3] and helpful in managing inflammatory and autoimmune diseases. Adding more omega-3 acid-rich foods to your diet is a worthwhile consideration. Some sources include cold-water fish (salmon, tuna, mackerel, herring, trout, anchovies, among others), nuts, seeds, plant oils, and dietary supplements.  Red meat

An extensive 2018 study found a link between increased consumption of red meat and endometriosis[4]. Women who ate two or more servings of red meat per day were 56% more likely to receive an endometriosis diagnosis (by laparoscopy) than those who consumed less than one serving per week.

One hypothesis for this finding is that red meat contains heme iron, which is associated with inflammation and oxidative stress mechanisms. So, reducing your intake of red meat may also reduce your endometriosis symptoms by lowering inflammation.

It's also worth noting women with endometriosis are frequently iron deficient, so it's worth discussing the role of red meat in your diet and your exact dietary needs with your health practitioner.

## Gluten

In one study, women with endometriosis were asked to cut out gluten for 12 months, and the results were encouraging. 75% of participants reported reduced pain when going gluten-free[5], and none reported any negative effects on their endometriosis.

## FODMAPs

Women with endometriosis are more likely to have irritable bowel syndrome (IBS), even when there is no endometriosis on the bowel. The two conditions can have overlapping symptoms.

A low FODMAP diet reduces the symptoms of IBS and may also do the same for endometriosis. Gluten is often found in the same foods high in FODMAPs, so by avoiding gluten, you can avoid some high FODMAP foods, too, and reduce endometriosis symptoms. However, if a gluten-free diet isn't significantly helping your symptoms, it maybe worth shifting to a low FODMAP diet to find relief like 72% of people did in this 2016 study.

Low FODMAP can be quite a restrictive diet, so it is important to review this option with your doctor and be monitored by a dietitian.

## Soy and soy-based products

Soybeans and soy products are high in estrogen and endometriosis is estrogen-dependent. However, researchers are still investigating the complete impact of eating soy on endometriosis. In one study, women given soy formula as infants had more than double the risk of endometriosis[7] compared with those who had never had soy formula at all.

**Caffeine and alcohol**

Health professionals recommend limiting your alcohol and coffee intake to lower inflammation and improve endometriosis. Coffee can also alter hormone levels, which may increase estrogen and worsen endometriosis. More clinical resea

## What Does Endometriosis Do to the Body?

Endometriosis is a chronic condition in which tissue similar to the lining of the uterus (endometrium) grows outside the uterus, commonly on the ovaries, fallopian tubes, outer surface of the uterus, and other pelvic organs. This misplaced tissue responds to hormonal changes during the menstrual cycle, causing inflammation, scarring, and pain. Here's how endometriosis affects the body:

1. Pain: The most common symptom of endometriosis is pelvic pain, which may vary in intensity and duration. It can occur before, during, or after menstruation, during intercourse, or during bowel movements or urination. The pain may also radiate to the lower back and legs.

2. Menstrual Irregularities: Endometriosis can cause irregular or heavy menstrual periods, as well as spotting between periods. Some individuals with endometriosis may experience infertility due to the scarring and distortion of pelvic anatomy.

3. Inflammation: The presence of endometrial-like tissue outside the uterus can trigger an inflammatory response in the body, leading to swelling, pain, and tissue damage.

4. Adhesions and Scarring: As endometriosis progresses, the repeated inflammation and healing cycles can result in the formation of scar tissue (adhesions) that may bind pelvic organs together, leading to pain and infertility.

5. Digestive Symptoms: Endometriosis can affect the digestive system, causing symptoms such as bloating, constipation, diarrhea, and nausea, particularly during menstruation.

6. Urinary Symptoms: In some cases, endometriosis may involve the bladder or ureters, leading to urinary symptoms such as urinary urgency, frequency, and pain during urination.

7. Fatigue: Chronic pain, hormonal imbalances, and associated symptoms of endometriosis can contribute to fatigue and decreased energy levels.

8. Emotional Impact: Living with chronic pain and the uncertainty of symptoms can take a toll on mental health, leading to anxiety, depression, stress, and impaired quality of life.

Endometriosis is a complex condition with varied symptoms and impacts on individual health. Early diagnosis and comprehensive management, including medical, surgical, and lifestyle interventions, can help alleviate symptoms and improve quality of life for individuals living with endometriosis.

# Chapter 6

# Alternative Therapies for Endometriosis

Alternative therapies offer additional options for managing endometriosis symptoms and promoting overall well-being. While they may not replace conventional medical treatments, many individuals find relief and support through complementary approaches. This chapter explores various alternative therapies that may complement traditional medical care for endometriosis.

1. Acupuncture:
Acupuncture, a traditional Chinese medicine practice, involves the insertion of thin needles into specific points on the body to stimulate energy flow and promote balance. Some studies suggest that acupuncture may help reduce pain and improve quality of life for individuals with endometriosis by modulating pain perception and reducing inflammation.

2. Herbal Medicine:
Herbal medicine, including herbal teas, supplements, and tinctures, is commonly used to alleviate symptoms associated with endometriosis. Certain herbs, such as turmeric, ginger, and chasteberry, have anti-inflammatory properties and may help reduce pain and inflammation. However, it's essential to consult with a qualified herbalist or healthcare provider before using herbal remedies, as they may interact with medications or have side effects.

3. Dietary Supplements:
Certain dietary supplements, such as omega-3 fatty acids, magnesium, and vitamin B6, may help alleviate endometriosis symptoms by reducing inflammation and supporting hormone balance. However, research on the efficacy of dietary supplements for endometriosis is limited, and their use should be discussed with a healthcare provider to ensure safety and effectiveness.

4. Mind-Body Therapies:
Mind-body therapies, including meditation, yoga, tai chi, and guided imagery, focus on the connection between the mind and body to promote relaxation,

reduce stress, and alleviate pain. These practices may help individuals with endometriosis manage pain, improve mood, and enhance overall well-being by fostering a sense of calm and control.

5. Pelvic Floor Therapy:
Pelvic floor physical therapy involves targeted exercises, manual techniques, and education to address pelvic floor dysfunction and alleviate pelvic pain associated with endometriosis. Pelvic floor therapy aims to improve pelvic muscle function, reduce tension, and restore mobility, providing relief from pain and discomfort.

Alternative therapies offer additional options for managing endometriosis symptoms and improving quality of life. While these approaches may not replace conventional medical treatments, they can complement traditional care and provide relief for some individuals. It's essential to work closely with a healthcare provider to develop a comprehensive treatment plan that incorporates both conventional and alternative therapies tailored to individual needs and preferences. Additionally, more research is needed to further explore the efficacy and safety of alternative therapies for endometriosis.

# Acupuncture and Traditional Chinese Medicine

Acupuncture and Traditional Chinese Medicine (TCM) have been used for centuries to treat various health conditions, including endometriosis. Here's how acupuncture and TCM approaches may help individuals with endometriosis:

## 1. Acupuncture:

Acupuncture involves the insertion of thin needles into specific points on the body to stimulate energy flow (Qi) and promote balance. It is believed that acupuncture can help regulate the body's energy pathways and address imbalances that contribute to symptoms like pain, inflammation, and hormonal disturbances associated with endometriosis. Some potential benefits of acupuncture for endometriosis include:

- Pain Relief: Acupuncture may help alleviate pelvic pain, menstrual cramps, and other types of pain associated with endometriosis by triggering the release of endorphins, the body's natural pain-relieving chemicals.

- Hormone Regulation: Acupuncture may help regulate hormonal imbalances by influencing the hypothalamic-pituitary-ovarian axis, which controls the menstrual cycle and hormone production.

- Stress Reduction: Acupuncture can promote relaxation and reduce stress levels, which may help manage the emotional and psychological impact of living with endometriosis.

2. Herbal Medicine:
Traditional Chinese herbal medicine is often used in conjunction with acupuncture to address underlying imbalances and promote healing. Herbal formulas may be prescribed based on individual symptoms, constitution, and patterns of disharmony identified through TCM diagnosis. Some herbs commonly used to treat endometriosis in TCM include:

- Dong Quai (Angelica sinensis): Known as the "female ginseng," dong quai is believed to regulate menstruation, relieve pain, and tonify blood.

- Chinese Peony (Paeonia lactiflora): Chinese peony is used to relieve menstrual pain, reduce inflammation, and promote blood circulation.

- Curcumin (Turmeric): Turmeric is a potent anti-inflammatory herb that may help alleviate pain and reduce inflammation associated with endometriosis.

3. Dietary Therapy:
TCM dietary therapy emphasizes the importance of maintaining a balanced diet to support overall health and address specific health concerns. In TCM, dietary recommendations for endometriosis may focus on promoting circulation, nourishing blood, and reducing dampness and heat. Some dietary guidelines for managing endometriosis in TCM may include:

- Consuming warming foods and spices like ginger, cinnamon, and garlic to improve circulation and alleviate cold and stagnation.

- Avoiding cold and damp-producing foods like dairy, sugar, and processed foods, which may exacerbate symptoms of stagnation and inflammation.

It's essential to consult with a licensed acupuncturist or TCM practitioner who has experience treating endometriosis to develop a personalized treatment plan tailored to your individual needs and preferences. While acupuncture and TCM can provide relief for some individuals with endometriosis, they are not a substitute for conventional medical treatment. It's important to work collaboratively with your healthcare team to address all aspects of your health and well-being.

## Aromatherapy and Essential Oils

Aromatherapy and essential oils are complementary therapies that involve the use of aromatic plant extracts to promote health and well-being. While research on the specific effects of aromatherapy and essential oils for endometriosis is limited, they may offer benefits in managing symptoms such as pain, stress, and inflammation. Here's how aromatherapy and essential oils may be used for endometriosis:

## 1. Pain Management:
Certain essential oils have analgesic properties and may help alleviate pelvic pain and menstrual cramps associated with endometriosis. Oils such as lavender, clary sage, chamomile, and marjoram are commonly used for their pain-relieving effects. These oils can be diluted in a carrier oil and applied topically to the abdomen or added to a warm bath for soothing relief.

## 2. Stress Reduction:
Living with endometriosis can be physically and emotionally taxing, leading to stress and anxiety. Aromatherapy can help promote relaxation and reduce stress levels. Essential oils like lavender, bergamot, ylang-ylang, and frankincense are known for their calming and mood-balancing effects. Diffusing these oils in the air or inhaling them directly can help induce feelings of relaxation and calm.

## 3. Anti-inflammatory Effects:
Endometriosis is characterized by inflammation, and certain essential oils possess anti-inflammatory

properties that may help alleviate symptoms. Oils such as frankincense, myrrh, turmeric, and ginger have anti-inflammatory properties and can be used topically or inhaled to reduce inflammation and pain associated with endometriosis.

4. Hormonal Balance:
Some essential oils are believed to have hormone-balancing effects, which may be beneficial for individuals with endometriosis. Oils like clary sage, geranium, and rose can help regulate hormone levels and support reproductive health. These oils can be used in aromatherapy blends or diluted in a carrier oil for topical application.

5. Emotional Support:
Living with chronic pain and managing the challenges of endometriosis can take a toll on mental health. Aromatherapy can provide emotional support and promote a sense of well-being. Essential oils like lavender, bergamot, rose, and jasmine are known for their mood-enhancing properties and can be used to uplift the spirits and promote a positive mindset.

It's important to use essential oils safely and consult with a qualified aromatherapist or healthcare provider, especially if you have any underlying health conditions or are pregnant. Essential oils should be properly diluted in a carrier oil before topical application to avoid skin irritation or sensitization. Additionally, individuals with asthma or respiratory conditions should use caution when inhaling essential oils, as strong aromas may trigger respiratory symptoms.

## Pelvic Physiotherapy and Yoga

Pelvic physiotherapy and yoga are two alternative therapies that can be beneficial for individuals with endometriosis. Here's how they can help:

1. Pelvic Physiotherapy:
Pelvic physiotherapy, also known as pelvic floor physical therapy, involves targeted exercises, manual therapy, and education to address pelvic floor dysfunction and alleviate pelvic pain and discomfort. For individuals with endometriosis, pelvic physiotherapy can help:

- Reduce Pelvic Pain: Pelvic physiotherapy techniques can help relieve pelvic pain by releasing muscle tension, improving blood flow, and restoring mobility to the pelvic area.

- Improve Pelvic Floor Function: Endometriosis can lead to pelvic floor dysfunction, including muscle tightness, weakness, and spasms. Pelvic physiotherapy can help strengthen and retrain the pelvic floor muscles to improve bladder and bowel function, reduce pain during intercourse, and support pelvic organ health.

- Enhance Mobility and Flexibility: Endometriosis-related pain and inflammation can restrict movement and flexibility in the pelvic area. Pelvic physiotherapy exercises and stretches can help improve mobility, reduce stiffness, and increase flexibility in the pelvic region.

2. Yoga:
Yoga is a mind-body practice that combines physical postures, breathwork, and meditation to promote relaxation, reduce stress, and improve overall well-being. For individuals with endometriosis, yoga can offer several benefits:

- Pain Relief: Certain yoga poses, such as gentle stretches, restorative poses, and poses that focus on opening the hips and pelvic area, can help alleviate pelvic pain and menstrual cramps associated with endometriosis.

- Stress Reduction: Endometriosis can be emotionally and mentally taxing, leading to stress and anxiety. Yoga practices, including mindfulness meditation, deep breathing exercises, and relaxation techniques, can help reduce stress levels and promote a sense of calm and balance.

- Hormonal Balance: Yoga practices that focus on gentle movement and breathwork can help regulate the endocrine system and promote hormonal balance, which may be beneficial for individuals with endometriosis.

- Improved Quality of Life: Engaging in regular yoga practice can improve overall quality of life for individuals with endometriosis by promoting physical, mental, and emotional well-being.

It's essential to work with a qualified pelvic physiotherapist or yoga instructor who has experience working with individuals with endometriosis to develop a tailored treatment plan that meets your specific needs and goals. Always listen to your body and modify exercises or poses as needed to avoid exacerbating symptoms. Additionally, consult with your healthcare provider before starting any new exercise or treatment regimen, especially if you have any underlying health conditions or concerns.

# Chapter 7

# Managing pain

Managing pain is a crucial aspect of coping with endometriosis and improving quality of life. Here are some strategies that may help alleviate pain associated with endometriosis:

1. Medications: Over-the-counter pain relievers such as nonsteroidal anti-inflammatory drugs (NSAIDs) like ibuprofen or naproxen can help reduce inflammation and alleviate menstrual cramps. Prescription medications, including hormonal contraceptives, progestins, or gonadotropin-releasing hormone (GnRH) agonists, may be recommended by a healthcare provider to manage pain and suppress endometriosis growth.

2. Heat Therapy: Applying heat to the lower abdomen or pelvic area can help relax muscles and alleviate pain. Use a heating pad, warm towel, or take a warm bath to soothe discomfort.

3. Exercise: Regular physical activity, such as walking, swimming, or yoga, can help improve

circulation, reduce stress, and release endorphins, which are natural pain relievers.

4. Dietary Changes: Some individuals find relief from endometriosis pain by making dietary modifications. Focus on a balanced diet rich in fruits, vegetables, whole grains, and lean proteins, and consider reducing consumption of inflammatory foods such as processed foods, refined sugars, and caffeine.

5. Stress Management: Practice relaxation techniques such as deep breathing, meditation, mindfulness, or guided imagery to reduce stress and promote relaxation, which can help alleviate pain.

6. Acupuncture and Acupressure: Traditional Chinese medicine modalities like acupuncture or acupressure may help relieve pain and promote overall well-being for some individuals with endometriosis.

7. Pelvic Floor Therapy: Pelvic floor physical therapy can help alleviate pelvic pain and dysfunction by addressing muscle tension, improving flexibility, and enhancing pelvic floor

function through specialized exercises and techniques.

8. Support Groups and Counseling: Joining a support group or seeking counseling can provide emotional support, validation, and coping strategies for managing the challenges of living with chronic pain and endometriosis.

It's essential to work closely with a healthcare provider to develop a personalized pain management plan tailored to your individual needs and preferences. This may involve a combination of treatments and lifestyle modifications to effectively manage pain and improve quality of life. Additionally, discuss any new or worsening symptoms with your healthcare provider to ensure appropriate evaluation and management.

## Can endometriosis go away on its own?

In some cases, endometriosis can go away on its own. Over time, endometriosis lesions can occasionally get smaller, and you may have fewer of them. This can also happen after menopause, which is often related to a drop in the amount of estrogen in your body.

For many people, endometriosis needs to be continuously treated to control symptoms like pain. It's important to maintain a regular appointment schedule with your healthcare provider so that you can work together on managing your condition long term.

## What happens if endometriosis is left untreated?

Over time, the endometrial-like tissue that grows outside of your uterus can cause cysts, adhesions and scar tissue. This can cause you to experience long-term (chronic) pain — especially during menstrual periods. Many people with endometriosis may also have difficulties getting pregnant. Treatment can sometimes help with this issue.

As you age and go through menopause, the symptoms of menopause may improve. This is related to the hormonal changes your body goes through during menopause.

# Chapter 8

# Lifestyle Modifications for Endo Wellness

There's no question that endometriosis can play havoc with your quality of life. In this condition, tissue that normally lines the uterus grows outside the uterus. Yet the ebb and flow of estrogen throughout the month works on this external endometrial tissue just as it does on the uterine lining, inciting growth when estrogen levels are high. That's fine for endometrial tissue within the uterus; but when endometrial tissue in the pelvic or abdominal cavity grows, it can cause severe pain, unusual bleeding and damage to other organs, including the bowel and bladder, and even lead to infertility. The pain can be so bad, in fact, that some women spend a day or more a month in bed.

While there are a variety of treatments for endometriosis—ranging from medications to surgery—you shouldn't discount lifestyle changes. We know that lifestyle changes, including what you eat and how much physical activity you get, affect other estrogen-dependent conditions, such as menstruation, fibroids and menopausal symptoms.

Unfortunately, the few studies on endometriosis and lifestyle focus on whether certain diets or levels of activity are connected to endometriosis, not whether those aspects improve endometriosis-related symptoms. However, that doesn't mean they're not worth a try.

Several studies find a strong connection between endometriosis and diets high in red meat and low in green vegetables and fresh fruit. This fits with other studies finding similar connections between these eating patterns and endometrial cancer and fibroids (noncancerous tumors of the uterus). One seminal study in this area compared 504 healthy women and 504 women with endometriosis, finding that women who ate beef every day were nearly twice as likely to have endometriosis, while those who got seven or more fruit and vegetable servings a week were at least 40 percent less likely.

So what's going on? One theory is that dietary fat influences your body's production of prostaglandins, chemicals that stimulate uterine contractions and affect ovarian functioning. It's thought that high levels of prostaglandins could lead to higher production of estrogen, which could influence the growth of endometrial tissue. Other studies find a link between high-fat diets and levels of circulating estrogen; the more fat in your diet, the more estrogen your body produces. This also occurs if you're overweight, and you're more likely to be overweight if you follow a diet high in red meat and low in fruits and vegetables.

Moving on to exercise, we know that women who exercise intensely tend to have lighter periods with reduced ovarian stimulation and estrogen production. In one study, researchers evaluated the effects of high-intensity physical activity on a woman's risk of endometriosis. They found that women who averaged 2.5 hours of high-intensity activity (think jogging, bicycling or aerobics) were 63 percent less likely to have endometriosis. Those who engaged in such activities more often were 76 percent less likely to be diagnosed with endometriosis.

## So what does this all mean to you?

Well, whether or not exercise and diet have any effect on endometriosis, we know they have a significant effect on a host of other health-related conditions. Reducing the amount of red meat in your diet, upping intake of fresh fruit and vegetables and getting three or more days of moderate- to high-high intensity exercise will help you in numerous ways—and may make a difference in the severity of your endometriosis. So they're certainly worth a try. Here are some ways to integrate both into your daily life:

- Stock the fridge with washed, precut veggies and fruit bowls. You're more likely to reach for something healthy if it's as easy to eat as that bag of chips.
- Build your meals around a vegetable course, not a meat course. Instead of pork chops with spinach on the side, sauté a huge amount of spinach and dice a bit of pork into it for the protein.
- Bump up the veggies and fruit in unexpected places. How about dicing zucchini and summer squash into your pasta sauce, topping salmon with a fruit salsa and mixing a bag of frozen broccoli into that mac and cheese or lasagna?
- Enlist a partner in your quest for exercise. Together, the two of you sign up for a class at

the gym, commit to brisk walking three mornings a week or agree to train for a 5-K run. It's much harder to skip out on a friend than it is to skip out on your own promise to exercise.

- Find something you love to do and do it! Who says exercise has to be a one-hour aerobics class at the gym or a solitary jog? How about signing up for Latina dance classes, creating a new garden, taking up racquetball or tennis, or learning to mountain bike?

## Pregnancy

**Will endometriosis symptoms get better or worse during pregnancy?**

Pregnancy may temporarily halt the painful periods and heavy menstrual bleeding that are often characteristic of endometriosis. It might provide some other relief as well.

Some people benefit by the increased levels of progesterone during pregnancy. It's thought that this hormone suppresses and perhaps even shrinks endometrial growths. In fact, progestin, a synthetic form of progesterone, is often used to treat those with endometriosis.

Other people, however, will find no improvement. You may even find that your symptoms worsen during pregnancy. That's because, as the uterus expands to accommodate the growing fetus, it can pull and stretch misplaced tissue. That can cause discomfort. An increase in estrogen can also feed endometrial growths.

Your experience during pregnancy may be different from other pregnant people with endometriosis. The severity of your condition, your body's hormone production, and the way your body responds to pregnancy will all affect how you feel.

Even if your symptoms do improve during pregnancy, they can resume after the birth of your baby. Breastfeeding may delay the return of symptoms, but once your period returns, your symptoms will likely return.

**Can you get pregnant if you have endometriosis?**

You can get pregnant if you have endometriosis. However, people with endometriosis can have a difficult time getting pregnant. This condition can be a common cause of infertility. If you have endometriosis and want to get pregnant, talk to your healthcare provider about the best treatment option for you. You might need to change your medication or, in some cases, pursue a surgical option to treat your endometriosis. Your provider will work with you to find the best treatment plan to help support a pregnancy.

## Risks and complications of pregnancy with endometriosis

Endometriosis may increase your risk for pregnancy and delivery complications. This may be caused by the inflammation, structural damage to the uterus, and hormonal influences endometriosis causes.

## Miscarriage
Several studies have documented that miscarriage rates are higher in those with endometriosis than in those without the condition. This holds true even for people with mild endometriosis.

One retrospective anal .ysis from 2017 concluded that people with endometriosis had a 35.8 percent chance of miscarriage versus 22 percent in those without the disorder. More research is needed to determine if endometriosis is a significant risk factor for miscarriage.

There's nothing you or your doctor can do to stop a miscarriage from happening, but it's important to recognize the signs so you can seek medical and emotional help to properly recover.

If you're fewer than 12 weeks pregnant, miscarriage symptoms resemble those of a menstrual period:

- bleeding
- cramping
- low back pain

You might also notice the passage of some tissue.

Symptoms after 12 weeks are mostly the same, but bleeding, cramping, and tissue passage might be more severe.

**Preterm birth**

According to an analysis of studies, pregnant people with endometriosis are 1.5 times more likely than other expectant moms to deliver before 37 weeks of gestation. A baby is considered preterm if he or she is born before 37 weeks of gestation.

Babies born prematurely tend to have a low birth weight and are more likely to experience health and developmental problems. Symptoms of early labor include:

- Regular contractions: Contractions are a tightening around your midsection, which may or may not hurt.
- Change in vaginal discharge: It may become bloody or the consistency of mucus.
- Pressure in your pelvis

If you're experiencing any of these symptoms, speak with your doctor. Early labor can sometimes cause, or be a symptom of your baby being in distress, and should be investigated to see if medical intervention is needed.

## Preterm birth

According to an analysis of studies, pregnant people with endometriosis are 1.5 times more likely than other expectant moms to deliver before 37 weeks of gestation. A baby is considered preterm if he or she is born before 37 weeks of gestation.

Babies born prematurely tend to have a low birth weight and are more likely to experience health and developmental problems. Symptoms of early labor include:

- Regular contractions: Contractions are a tightening around your midsection, which may or may not hurt.
- Change in vaginal discharge: It may become bloody or the consistency of mucus.
- Pressure in your pelvis

If you're experiencing any of these symptoms, speak with your doctor. Early labor can sometimes cause, or be a symptom of your baby being in distress, and should be investigated to see if medical intervention is needed.

**Placenta previa**
During pregnancy, a foetus and placenta will develop. The placenta supplies oxygen and nourishment to your growing fetus through your blood.

Most placentas attach to the uterine walls, away from the cervix. However, in some, the placenta may be close to or directly on the opening to the cervix. This is known as placenta previa.

Placenta previa can increase your risk for significant bleeding and placenta abruption — a premature and dangerous separation of the placenta from the uterus.

People with endometriosis may be at increased risk for this life-threatening condition. The main symptom is bright red vaginal bleeding. If the bleeding is minimal, you may be advised to limit your activities, including sex and exercise. If bleeding is heavy, you may need a blood transfusion and an emergency C-section.

# Conclusion

Endometriosis is a common, estrogen-dependent, chronic gynecological disorder. It is characterized by the presence of uterine endometrial tissue outside the uterine cavity. Endometriosis may present as superficial and/or deep pelvic peritoneal implants, adhesions, and ovarian cysts (endometriomas). The symptoms of endometriosis include pelvic pain and infertility. Affected women are at higher risk than the general population for developing fibromyalgia, chronic fatigue syndrome, autoimmune inflammatory diseases, and atopic diseases. The association between endometriosis and stress is an intriguing but poorly investigated issue. However, it is possible that endometriosis may be associated with the dysregulation of the stress system. Endometriosis requires multidisciplinary care and long-term follow-ups for the surveillance of associated disorders that may develop in susceptible women.

**Can you still have endometriosis after menopause?**

Menopause is a time of major change in your body. One thing that happens during this transition is a change in the levels of hormones in your body, specifically estrogen. There's a link between your reproductive hormones and endometriosis. After menopause, with decreased estrogen levels, endometriosis lesions often decrease. This can also mean that you no longer experience symptoms of the condition or that they're less intense than before menopause.

However, if you take hormones as a treatment for any symptoms you experience during menopause, your endometriosis may still cause symptoms.

www.ingramcontent.com/pod-product-compliance
Lightning Source LLC
Chambersburg PA
CBHW061648250726
48659CB00004B/1419